YOUR KNOWLEDGE HAS VALUE

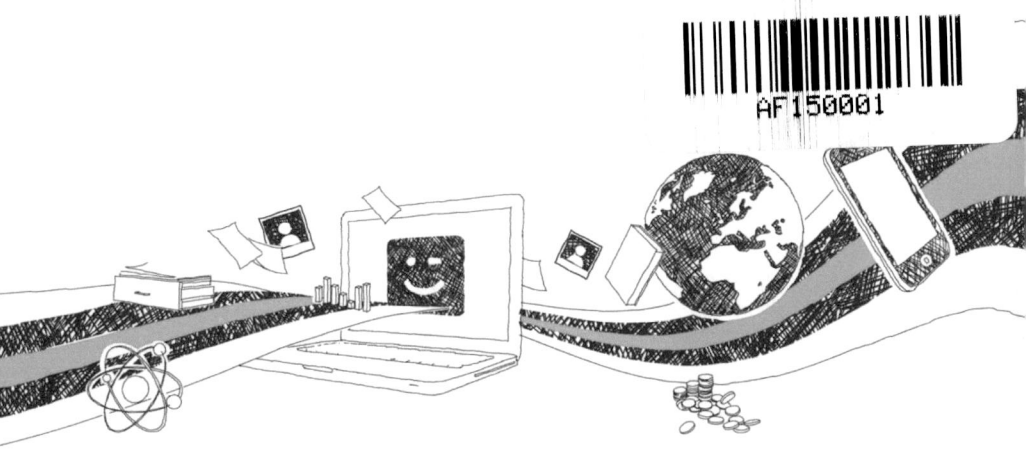

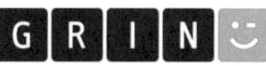

Richards Macdonald

Metal Health In Australia

GRIN Publishing

Bibliographic information published by the German National Library:

The German National Library lists this publication in the National Bibliography; detailed bibliographic data are available on the Internet at http://dnb.dnb.de .

Imprint:

Copyright © 2011 GRIN Verlag GmbH
Print and binding: Books on Demand GmbH, Norderstedt Germany
ISBN: 978-3-656-41694-4

This book at GRIN:

http://www.grin.com/en/e-book/213352/metal-health-in-australia

GRIN - Your knowledge has value

Since its foundation in 1998, GRIN has specialized in publishing academic texts by students, college teachers and other academics as e-book and printed book. The website www.grin.com is an ideal platform for presenting term papers, final papers, scientific essays, dissertations and specialist books.

Visit us on the internet:

http://www.grin.com/

http://www.facebook.com/grincom

http://www.twitter.com/grin_com

Mental health in Australia

Introduction

Public health systems have an aim of aiding in the prevention of diseases in a country. Many diseases affect the society some of which are non-infectious chronic diseases, while others are infectious. Some of the diseases affect majority of the population in certain countries.Mental health is usually described as the way in which individuals feel, think or act as they cope with life situations. It is very important to stay mentally healthy through every stage of life. Mental illness may be as a result of disorders which are common. This paper will discuss the health care system in Australia in regard to mental health as a major concern.

Discussion

Statistics on the effect of mental health illness in Australia

More than 20% of Australians suffer from mental illness at least ones in their lives. Some suffer from more than one form of the same. Around 20000 Australians are diagnosed of mental illness annually which raises concern within the health system. At least three million out of these get depressive illness while five percent suffer from anxiety. Others suffer from schizophrenia while others go through serious psychotic illnesses (1).

There have been surveys done showing that one in every five Australians is affected by mental illness. In this category, women report more on cases of anxiety and affective disorders than men. Men however, are more likely to have disorders that are as a result of substance abuse such as alcohol. They are also more prone to schizophrenia .It has also been noted that compulsive disorders are very common in both sexes with at least 90% of eating disorders occurring among women (2).

Populations most affected by mental illness are around the ages of 18 to 24 with at least 14% of children below 17years being affected by problems of mental health (2). Conditions such as schizophrenia and bipolar disorders however occur after teenage hood with adolescents exhibiting use of drugs or high rate of suicidal thoughts. It has been noted that culture affects the access to medication since those individuals from diverse cultural backgrounds can't access health services as often as those in the mainstream population

(2).Mental health illnesses have been shown to be the main cause of absenteeism in the work place in Australia. It is estimated that at least six million days of working are lost each year due to cases resulting from mental health illnesses. It makes up at least 30% of disability claims in the country which translates to $15 annually (2). It has also been observed that disability or acquiring of other disorders can increase the chances of suicide and depression in people who are older and come from diverse cultural backgrounds. It is estimated that in 2003-2004, mental health accounted for 12% of the days spent in hospital by patients' (3). The diagnosis for depressive disorders amounted to around 36% of hospitalizations while schizophrenia recorded the highest number of separations being 11% (3).

No difference has been found while comparing populations in the rural areas and those who live in the urban parts of Australia in regards to mental health. Research however, has revealed that males in the urban areas suffer more from mental illnesses as a result of substance use. Most people have misconceptions about mental health due to low education or inadequate information. Some believe that those who are mentally ill are violent yet as research has shown those with mental disorders usually have no history of violent behavior (2). It is also misconceived that mental illness cannot be cured yet it has been observed that most people suffering from it recover quickly if they get medicated on time. There are various forms of mental illnesses and these affect people across diverse cultures.

Types of mental problems

A number of mental disorders are common in Australia and anxiety disorder is one of them. Those suffering from anxiety disorders dread certain objects or situations and respond with nervousness. Anxiety disorder is easily diagnosed if the individual's reaction to a situation is not appropriate. Anxiety could thus cause interference with the individual's normal functioning. Various forms include post traumatic stress, generalized anxiety, social anxiety disorder, obsessive-compulsive disorder and panic disorders (4). Certain phobias may also be included in the list. Mental illness could also take the form of mood disorders. These include depression, mania and bipolar disorders. These disorders may result to suicidal and self harm tendencies if untreated.

Psychotic disorders are also a common occurrence in the Australian population. They involve distorted thinking and awareness. Hallucinations are one form of psychotic disorder and occur when the individual sees images or hears sounds that are not real (4). It is mainly influenced by substance abuse or other diseases that affect the brain.

Eating disorders such as anorexia nervosa, bulimia nervosa and binge eating disorders are also considered as mental illnesses as they involve a lot of emotion and have a great impact on the individual's life. Bulimia itself, involves bingeing on food then purging and can lead to gum disease, osteoporosis, heart disease, kidney disease or death (5).Others suffer from impulse control and addiction disorders such as kleptomania which is an impulse to steal, and pyromania a compulsion to start fires, which all pose harm to the individual and others(4). These compulsions are also usually accompanied by use of drugs.

Factors that cause mental illnesses

There are a number of factors that lead to development of mental illnesses. One of them is genetics. Scientific research, has shown that mental illness is sometimes an inherited condition and may affect an individual if some one in the family also suffers from the same(6). In most cases, it is usually dormant and is triggered by a number of factors such as stress, abuse, or traumatic events.

Some infections can also lead to mental illness by causing brain damage. An example is infection by streptococcus bacteria leading to pediatric autoimmune neuropsychiatry disorder which affects children (7).Brain injury through accidents may also result in mental illness. Treatment should be sought for all injuries on the head to avoid such complications.

Prenatal disruption of the brain development has also been shown to be a cause for the mental illnesses witnessed in Australia. Autism is said to be caused by poor flow of oxygen to the brain of the developing fetus (8). Another factor is poor nutrition as a result of poverty or intake of drugs. Psychological factors such as trauma in childhood, neglect, early loss of parents and sexual abuse have all been shown to have an effect on the mental health of an individual. Environmental factors such as cultural expectations have also been shown to cause metal illness when the individual is under pressure or stress.

Intake of drugs such as alcohol, smoking, and use of hallucinogens has also been a major factor contributing to mental illness in the population. Some of these drugs are illegal and the consequences of using them lead to adverse brain damage as individuals become dependent on the drugs the individuals may thus find it hard to seek help as the continue in the use of the drugs(8) .This is usually the case among the young adults and teenagers. The result is that the individual begins having memory loss, hallucinations, and may even die as a result of the same.

Effect of mental illness in society

Public health services focus on the improvement of health for the whole country and not just for individuals. In this regard, the public healthcare system has been given the role of raising awareness on the determinants of mental health. It has also been given a role of reporting and monitoring environmental conditions and social trends that determine mental health. Health care systems have also been given the mandate to coordinate public health planning. Mental health affects the education sector as people suffering from various illnesses find it hard to cope in schools especially when they are picked on or bullied by their fellow students. It may lead to feelings of depression, self harm and suicide as the individual tries to get away from the situation (8). This has led to numerous dropouts of students with some of them acquiring habits of drug abuse as they try to cope with situations. The parents and teachers in most cases are unaware of the conditions affecting the students.

There is stigma associated with mental illness and as a result most individuals avoid seeking help from health centers. Some who suffer from self harm find it difficult to report their condition for fear of hospitalization in mental facilities or arrest incase their condition is related to intake of illegal drugs (9). This further leads to stress on the part of their friends and families who may be worried about their condition. Incase the individual dies out of suicide; it could lead to some of the family members or friends acquiring a stress related mental illness.

Actions taken to improve mental health and limitations

In 2002, a health action plan was developed that talks of the government vision for health .It envisions a health system that is inclusive and fair while being committed to the protection of the vulnerable and those in need (10). It states that individuals should access quality services in order to meet their needs. Priority for all actions regarding health, target the vulnerable and those with poor economic status. These are the principles outlined in the health action plan. Health action plan also refers to the world health organization document on social determinants of health and states that the government approach towards health should address the social determinants in order to ensure equity (10). It thus talks of reducing health in equality by providing it to all.

A mental health system which is effective requires funding in order to develop policies and train experts. Funding would be used to undertake research and maintain facilities. According to the world health organization, there are many things that need to be addressed in Australia's health system. One of these issues is the lack of specialists mental illness care. The health policy in Australia has not addressed the shortage of staff in hospitals and health centers dealing with mental problems. Specialists such as psychiatrists and nurses are very few in number compared to the population that requires their services (11). There are very few of those being trained in these specialized fields which creates a problem of lack of adequate personnel to handle mental cases.

There is also a form of discrimination in hospitalization. Australia has a policy of rationing its medical services to the public especially when it comes to mental illness (11).Criteria used allows only cases that are extreme to be hospitalized while those that are less extreme are discharged early or not admitted at all(11). This does not allow them to receive proper treatment for their conditions.

Another problem involved with the Australian health system is that it does not allow the publishing of living conditions of the carers and patients (11). This is a form of cover up to avoid accountability when dealing with mental illness. It also creates a problem when patients who are mentally ill are put in the same ward as those undergoing geriatric care as this is a reflection of over-generalized treatment. When patients don't receive specialized care in hospitals, it discourages them from going to hospital again.

Suggestions to improve the mental health system

In 2010, the national health and hospitals network agreement was approved at the council of Australian Governments meeting. It had three objectives one of which was to reform the fundamentals of Australian health system through funding and change of governance in order to be in a position to offer better services (12). It also addressed the aspect of changing service delivery in the health sector by making integrated care more accessible to patients (12). It addressed the need to improve the infrastructure in hospitals and hire more doctors and nurses. This agreement however, did not change much in health care regarding mental health as out of the $7.4billion that had been expected to reform the sector; only $181.3 was directed to mental health (12).

After a forum held recently, a number of issues were raised that affect the people suffering from mental illness. One of them is the stigma against those with mental illness together with their carers and the discrimination they face (12). Another issue raised was considering the minority groups such as linguistically different people with different cultures suffering from mental illness. A few things are missing from the governments overall policy for reforming the health sector. These include consumer and carer participation, employment, housing, mental health work force, a mental health promotion, an anti-stigma campaign and a life course approach to early prevention (12).

When it comes to consumer and carer participation, Australia doesn't have the required structures to enable their participation in the delivery of services dealing with mental health. Recruitment should be carried out targeting people from a variety of backgrounds including those in the rural areas as well as those in the urban ones. Different cultures should also be incorporated in the recruitment so as to adequately represent the views of the majority as well as minorities in implementation of policy (12). This will help in making the health system more flexible to meet the patient's needs.

Housing is another factor that needs improvement. This is because it stands out as one of the main obstacles to the lives of people suffering from mental illness. This is because recovering from a mental related illness without adequate housing is almost impossible. The 2009 MHCA publication, points out some observations on housing (12). One of the observations is that those who suffer from mental illness and lack adequate housing are likely to become unwell and would hence require being hospitalized (12). MHCA publication also points out that acute mental illness makes individuals more prone to homelessness. Those who can obtain accommodation of their choice it was observed, feel more in control and less stressed. Despite these recommendations there has been little done to improve the conditions of living for the mentally ill.

It is also important to address the issue of employment of those suffering from mental conditions .This is because it helps in the quick recovery of a patient when working on something he or she likes. This is because work in most cases empowers the individual which is very important as the person suffering from mental illness should always be at the centre control of his or her life (12). Rate of employment of people among those with disability in Australia is however, very low and more needs to be done by the government to address this problem.

Early intervention of mental illness could help reduce complications that result from advanced illness. These interventions should include both the clinical aspects and other social determinants. There should be programs that deal with infants to ensure that any mental health issue is detected and treated early enough (12). Early intervention will also save the costs incurred in the long term medication of an individual.

In Australia, there is still misinformation among the public when it comes to mental illness. This has resulted to stigmatization of those affected and discrimination in the work place and social circles. Disorders such as schizophrenia and bipolar disorders face negative stigma from the community and the media (12). It is therefore important, that the government undertakes campaigns to promote mental health and reduce the stigma that surrounds it. This will help to give people information on how to manage the risk factors causing mental illness. It will also help to pass information on the importance of early intervention and ways in which individuals can avoid relapses.

It is also important to have a mental work force that is well trained to handle cases of mental illness. With the current shortage in staff, dealing with mental illness such as psychiatrists, nurses, and general practitioners, more needs to be done to recruit staff in hospitals especially in the rural areas (12). More information should be given to trainees as it is believed that the stigma surrounding mental health illnesses is a reason for the low level of health practitioners interested in the field. With an adequate working force, the health system would be better equipped to deal with the mental health crisis. Ottawa charter has been helpful in promoting health policies as it highlights importance of creating a healthy public policy, a supportive environment, strengthening of community action, development of personal skills and reorientation of health services (13). If the policies are used as a whole in a public setting or in a community, they are likely to promote health rather than when only some of the policies are used. Ottawa charter further outlines the role of organizations, communities, systems and individuals in strategies to promote health (14).

In 1997, four aspects of mental health promotion were tabulated. These included promoting positive mental health, primary prevention, early recognition, intervention and treatment and rehabilitation of mental disorders and problems. These principles were in line with the Ottawa charter that gives directions on the way forward when dealing with health issues (14). The strategies were meant to help people increase their control on mental health, prevent depression, and avoid the development of antisocial behavior (14).

Inspire foundation is one of the organizations that was formed to deal with mental illness among the young people. It was formed as a reaction to the high number of suicides among the youth and has its goals linked with the objectives and principles of the Ottawa Charter. One of its goals is to develop personal skills by increasing mental health literacy of young people (15). It also creates supportive environments by reducing the stigma related to mental illness. Inspire foundation also strengthens community action by providing teachers with confidence to address students on strategies to prevent mental illness.

Inspire foundation also reorients health services by recognizing the role played by technology in the lives of young people and using the same to offer psychological support and mental health care (15). It also helps the young people in advocating for better mental health policies. Through information, it offers the society of those that are mentally ill access to comfort and hence quicker recovery. This in turn reduces the number of people and youth who lose their lives as a result of suicide.

It is important to note that mental health is highly dependent on the policies operating at all levels of society. In order to have a sound mental health policy, there is need to acquire resources and address the causes for the mental illnesses (16). Issues such as poverty, racism, unemployment, and violence need to be addressed as they form a significant root cause for some of the mental illnesses (17). It should also be clear that in order to deal with the problems of mental health, more needs to be understood on the causes that lead to the same.

It is important to take a number of steps to promote development of mental health in the country. One of the steps is to implement broad population measures by creating awareness and destigmatisation of the public (18, 19). There should also be a rapid expansion of health care services that deal with the youth as they are most affected by mental illness (20). Depression treatments should be made available through primary care with early intervention programs being put in place (21).

Development of programs that deal with health care of young people should incorporate measures, to deal with first episodes of mental illness (22, 23). This will help in prevention of a relapse once the patient is healed (24). A workforce should also be in place to deal with psychiatric disorders (25). Government hospitals furthermore, should be made accountable in terms of providing affordable medical care for the patient having mental health problems (16). Standards of care should also be maintained for those handling cases of mental illness. This will ensure that the patients recover quickly as they are given more attention by the healthcare workers.

Conclusion

In conclusion, mental health is an issue of great significance to the Australian public health system. Actions taken to promote mental health are still below what is expected as per the Ottawa charter. More needs to be done to reduce the stigma associated with the mental illness. Patients who suffer from mental illnesses and disorders should also be given adequate information on how best to handle their conditions. Some of the potential barriers to the success of mental health promotion include ignorance on the part of government officials charged with the mandate to implement health policy and failure of individuals to seek help in hospitals for their illnesses. Government commitment in terms of funding is also a hindrance to the improvement of services offered to patients suffering from mental illness.

Community programs that offer support to individuals through sports and other events should be formed to support people in the community undergoing mental health problems. This will create a forum whereby people can share their experiences and in this way encourage each other. Home based care should also be introduced for individuals who for certain reasons cannot access the hospital. This will go a long way in avoiding complications that result from untreated mental illnesses.

References

1. Hunter Institute of mental health .Overview of mental illness in Australia. Common wealth of Australia [Internet] 2009. [Cited 2011, May 25].Available from http://www.responseability.org/site/index.cfm?display=134563

2. Mind frame media initiative. Mental illness facts. Media professionals [Internet] 2011. [Cited 2011, May 25].Available from http://www.mindframe-media.info/site/index.cfm?display=86529

3. Australian bureau of statistics. Mental health in Australia: A snapshot 2004-2005.[Internet] December 30, 2006. [Cited 2011, May 25].Available from http://www.abs.gov.au/ausstats/abs@.nsf/mf/4824.0.55.001

4. Web MD. Types of mental illness. Mental health. [Internet] May 25, 2011. [Cited 2011, May 25].Available from http://www.webmd.com/mental-health/mental-health-types-illness

5. Web MD. Bulimia nervosa. Bulimia nervosa health centre. [Internet] May 25, 2011. [Cited 2011, May 25].Available from http://www.webmd.com/mental-health/bulimia-nervosa/default.htm

6. Mayo Clinic. Mental illness risk factors.[Internet]. September 1, 2010. [Cited 2011, May 25].Available from http://www.mayoclinic.com/health/mental-illness/DS01104/DSECTION=risk-factors

7. Web MD. Causes of mental illness .Anxiety and panic disorders health centre. [Internet] May 25, 2011. [Cited 2011 May 25, 2011].Available from http://www.webmd.com/anxiety-panic/mental-health-causes-mental-illness

8. Southern public health unit network. Social determinants of health. [Internet]. [Cited 2011, May 25].Available from http://www.health.qld.gov.au/ph/Documents/saphs/20402.pdfs

9. Newman L, Baum F, and Harris E.Summary for the Australian Capital Territory. Australian government and health Inequities project. [Internet].2003. [Cited 2011, May 25].Available from http://som.flinders.edu.au/FUSA/PublicHealth/AHIP/Goverments%20and%20Health%20Inequities%20Project/ACT%20Summary.pdf

10. Adrienne G.Who's healthy? Mental illness in Australia compared to around the world. Mental health foundation ACT. [Internet] 2009. [Cited 2011, May 25].Available from http://www.mhf.org.au/mhf/awareness.aspx?a=18&s=99&c=296

11. Mental health council of Australia. Out of hospital out of mind. [Internet]. April, 2003. [Cited 2011, May 25].Available from http://www.mhca.org.au/Publications/documents/OutofHospitalOutofMindReport.pdf

12. Mental health council of Australia. Priorities outside the NHHN reforms. [Internet]. [Cited 2011, May 25].Available from http://www.mhca.org.au/documents/submissions/MHCA%20Position%20Paper%202%20-%20Priorities%20outside%20the%20NHHN%20reforms.pdf

13. Bernadette W, Glenda V.Young people and alcohol misuse: how nurses can use the Ottawa Charter for health promotion. Australian journal of advanced nursing volume 25 number 4. [Internet]. [Cited 2011, May 25].Available from http://www.ajan.com.au/Vol25/Vol_25-4_Ward.pdf

14. Epidemiol community health. Promoting mental health: Recent progress and problems in Australia. [Internet].2000. [Cited 2011, May 25].Available from http://www.ncbi.nlm.nih.gov/pmc/articles/PMC1731617/pdf/v054p00082.pdf

15. Inspire foundation. The Ottawa charter in action. [Internet]. [Cited 2011, May 25].Available from

http://hsc.csu.edu.au/pdhpe/core1/focus/focus1_3/4015/health_pri1_4_1_4_inspire.ht
m

16. Ian BH, Grace LG, Patrick DM, Tracey AD and Georgina ML.Australian mental health reform: time for real outcomes. [Internet].MJA 2005. [Cited 2011, May 25].Available from http://www.mja.com.au/public/issues/182_08_180405/hic10810_fm.html

17. WHO European ministerial conference. Mental health: facing the challenges, building solutions. [Internet]. [Cited 2011, May 25].Available from http://www.euro.who.int/__data/assets/pdf_file/0008/96452/E87301.pdf

18. Council of social services. National health reform-outcomes of the 29th council of Australian governments meeting. [Internet]. May 2010. [Cited 2011, May 25].Available from http://www.ncoss.org.au/resources/100511-NCOSS-Briefing-paper-on-COAG-NHHN-Agreement-20-April-2010.pdf

19. Mental health council. CoAG must drastically increase its funding. MHCA media release [Internet].April 15, 2011. [Cited 2011, May 25].Available from http://connetica.com.au/_webapp_829736/MHCA_Media_Release

20. Australian medical association. NHHRC report and COAG reforms. Psychiatrist's newsletter. [Internet]. April 2010. [Cited 2011, May 25].Available from http://ama.com.au/node/5528

21. Common wealth of Australia. Common wealth response to the hidden toll: Suicide in Australia report of the senate community affairs reference committee. [Internet].2010. [Cited 2011, May 25].Available from http://www.health.gov.au/internet/mentalhealth/publishing.nsf/content/9DCC6D6FD C295C1ECA2577B5007B77B3/$File/D0188%20Doc%20-%20Commonwealth%20Response%20to%20The%20Hidden%20Toll%20Suicide%2 0In%20Australia%20%20PRINT_Revisions161210.pdf

22. Health issues centre. Health reform. [Internet]. [Cited 2011, May 25].Available from http://www.healthissuescentre.org.au/subjects/list-library-subject.chtml?subject=11

23. Parliament of Australia. National health and hospitals Network bill. [Internet].Released August 2008. [Cited 2011, May 25].Available from http://parlinfo.aph.gov.au/parlInfo/search/display/display.w3p;query=BillId_Phrase% 3A%22r4433%22%20Dataset%3Abillsdgs;rec=0

24. Health workforce. National health workforce Innovation and reform strategy frame work for action [Internet]. [Cited 2011, May 25].

25. Victorian Government .Because mental health matters. Consultation paper. [Internet]May 2008. [Cited 2011, May 25].Available from http://www.health.vic.gov.au/mentalhealth/reformstrategy/documents/mhmatters-rep08.pdf